ACE Group F

Fitness Yoga

by Mara Carrico

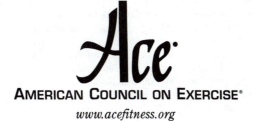

AMERICAN COUNCIL ON EXERCISE®
www.acefitness.org

Library of Congress Catalog Card Number: 00-104274

First edition
ISBN 1-890720-05-4
Copyright © 2000 American Council on Exercise® (ACE®)
Printed in the United States of America.

All rights reserved. Except for use in a review, the reproduction or utilization of this work in any form or by any electronic, mechanical, or other means, now known or hereafter invented, including xerography, photocopying and recording, and in any information retrieval system, is forbidden without the written permission of the American Council on Exercise.

A B C D E F

Distributed by:
American Council on Exercise
P. O. Box 910449
San Diego, CA 92191-0449
(858) 535-8227
(858) 535-1778 (FAX)
www.acefitness.org

Managing Editor: Daniel Green
Design: Karen McGuire
Production: Glenn Valentine
Manager of Publications: Christine Ekeroth
Associate Editor: Joy Keller
Index: Bonny McLaughlin
Models: Steve Paredes and Corinne LaReau

Acknowledgements:
Thanks to the entire American Council on Exercise staff for their support and guidance through the process of creating this manual.

NOTICE
The fitness industry is ever-changing. As new research and clinical experience broaden our knowledge, changes in programming and standards are required. The authors and the publisher of this work have checked with sources believed to be reliable in their efforts to provide information that is complete and generally in accord with the standards accepted at the time of publication. However, in view of the possibility of human error or changes in industry standards, neither the authors nor the publisher nor any other party who has been involved in the preparation or publication of this work warrants that the information contained herein is in every respect accurate or complete, and they are not responsible for any errors or omissions or the results obtained from the use of such information. Readers are encouraged to confirm the information contained herein with other sources.

REVIEWERS

Molly Fox has been training students and instructors in fitness, dance, and yoga for approximately 20 years. As former owner and operator of New York City–based Molly Fox Studios, she received the Fitness Businessperson of the Year Award from IDEA. Fox has written numerous books, been featured in videos, and served as a consultant for top fitness companies. Currently, Fox is owner of Yoga People™, a yoga center in Brooklyn, NY, fitness consultant to Equinox Fitness Clubs in Manhattan, and program designer/choreographer for Body Training Systems and The Step Co.

Leslie Ferree, certified yoga instructor in the Indri Devi Method, has taught yoga for more than 25 years. She instructs classes and trains teachers in the classical style appropriate for all levels. Ferree established the Camelrock Yoga Center in Valley Center, Calif., to bring people together to practice yoga, experience relaxing retreats, and benefit from wellness workshops.

TABLE OF CONTENTS

Introduction		...ix
Chapter One	Introduction To Fitness Yoga	...1
	History	*Benefits*
	Growth	*Styles of Hatha Yoga*
Chapter Two	Teaching A Yoga Class	...8
	Equipment	*Personal Limitations*
	Environment	*Modifications*
	Music	*Exercise Leadership*
Chapter Three	Basic Asana Repertoire	...14
	Standing Poses	*Supine Poses*
	Balancing Posture	*Inverted Pose*
	Seated Poses	*Sun Salutation*
	Prone Poses	*SIDEBAR: Power Yoga*
Chapter Four	Breath Awareness	...44
	Breath Awareness Techniques (Pranayama)	
Chapter Five	Programming	...46
	Frequency of Practice	*Contraindications /*
	Components	*High-risk Poses*
	Safety Rules	*Intensity Monitoring*
	Injury Prevention	*SIDEBAR: Controversial Poses*
Chapter Six	Yoga Teacher Standards And Certification	...55
Glossary		...56
Index		...59
References and Suggested Reading		...64

INTRODUCTION

The American Council on Exercise (ACE) is pleased to include *Fitness Yoga* as a Group Fitness Specialty Book. As the industry continues to expand, evolve, and redefine itself, yoga is increasingly recognized as a viable component of fitness. It has also become apparent that guidelines and criteria should be established so that yoga, as a fitness activity, can be practiced both safely and beneficially. The intent of this book is to educate and give guidance to fitness professionals who wish to teach yoga. As with all areas of fitness, education is a continual process. ACE recognizes that yoga is a broad subject requiring serious study. Therefore, we have included teaching and certification standards as established within the yoga community itself.

Chapter One

Introduction to Fitness Yoga

Yoga as an exercise activity has become a permanent fixture in the fitness arena. Long recognized as an effective stress-management technique and a great way to improve flexibility, **yoga** has more recently become known for what it can do for building strength and stamina. Yoga classes have become a standard feature of class schedules in gyms, health clubs, and spas. HMOs often include discounts to yoga classes for policyholders, while many hospitals offer yoga as part of both rehabilitation and community outreach programs. This popularity has been a contributing factor to the growth in mind-body exercise, which continues to be an increasingly important part of the industry. As a result, qualified instructors are in demand.

Yoga, however, is much more than another form of exercise. It is part of an extensive ancient East Indian philosophical tradition. What we refer to as "yoga" — the exercise activity — is really **hatha yoga**, the physical aspect of this philosophy. There are many different ways in which hatha may be practiced. Guidelines govern the practice and reflect the basic principles of yoga, regardless of style. It takes education, maturity, and experience to teach yoga safely and effectively.

History

Yoga is believed to be a 5,000-year-old philosophy orally transmitted from teacher to student. The Indian sage Patanjali is credited with putting this tradition into writing approximately 2,000 years ago in his classic work, *The Yoga Sutras*. This treatise dispenses direction concerning all levels of human potential: physical, mental, emotional, and spiritual. It provides guidance on personal development that includes standards for ethical and moral conduct.

Hatha yoga, initially created to prepare the body for **meditation**, is an important part of this process. The technique includes exercises designed to strengthen the body and nervous system, thereby creating the appropriate psychophysiological state for a higher level of consciousness. The repertoire consists of postures, movements, breathing, and relaxation techniques that affect every system of the body, bringing about an optimal state of health and well-being.

You will undoubtedly encounter questions regarding yoga's religious and spiritual components. When you do, stress that yoga is not a religion. However, its philosophy has been embraced by religious traditions in India and elsewhere. In fact, the foundations of yoga are congruent with the tenets of all the great religions of the world. Practicing hatha yoga and embracing the philosophy of yoga will not interfere with any belief system that supports the intrinsic value of all living things or religious inclination that addresses the existence of a higher power.

Growth

Although yoga's appearance in the West is rather recent, its roots can be traced to mid-nineteenth-century America. At that time, the transcendentalist authors Ralph Waldo Emerson and Henry David Thoreau were deeply inspired by Hindu texts and are credited with planting the seeds for yoga's growth in America. Primarily embraced for its spiritual elements by a relatively small and elite portion of the populace, hatha yoga did not emerge as a fitness option until the 1950s. Even then, its health benefits were appreciated by relatively few people for another 25 to 30 years.

Yoga's current status reflects the growing interest in the **mind-body connection**. Continuing research in both the medical and fitness communities supports the important role the mind plays in promoting wellness, reducing stress, and combating disease. Yoga techniques provide both a blueprint for stress management and a system for physical fitness. There is also a therapeutic aspect to the practice of yoga. This area deals with specific breathing techniques, poses, and meditations to remedy various structural, physiological, and psychological conditions.

Whereas fitness experts once paid little attention to what yoga had to offer, leaders in the field now recognize its value as a viable fitness choice. While not all styles of hatha cover all the essential facets of a fitness regimen — aerobic, strength, and flexibility training — many do. At the very least, hatha yoga can provide a balanced strength and flexibility workout that can be supplemented with a cardiovascular routine.

Fitness options for the burgeoning baby-boomer market will be of paramount importance as we move into the new millennium. The popularity of safe and effective mind-body exercises will create a need for a growing number of qualified instructors.

Benefits

Yoga offers many benefits. While the ultimate goal of this age-old philosophy is to realize our divine nature, the positive effects on physical health and mental well-being are impressive. Hatha yoga's methodology dictates a balance between effort and relaxation and positively influences every system of the body. The repertoire includes poses for strength, flexibility, and balance. Some styles even include a cardiovascular component. The breathing techniques in yoga improve respiration while producing a cognitive quiescence, or "mental stillness," and an associated decrease in central nervous system activity. In fact, the breathing and meditative techniques of yoga, long known as effective stress and pain management tools, have been employed by Western physicians and therapists for a good portion of the 20th century. Many modern day methods such as biofeedback and Dr. Herbert Benson's Relaxation Response (Benson, 1976) are patterned after these techniques.

In addition to promoting strength and flexibility, it is believed that yoga can promote healing if practiced under supervision in a controlled fashion.

Styles of Hatha Yoga

As indicated earlier, there are many different styles, or systems, of hatha practice. Some are vigorous and intense while others are gentle and more meditative. While yoga itself is a very ancient practice, most of the hatha systems practiced today have been refined and developed in the twentieth century. You should be aware of newly emerging hybrids of these systems, developed by teachers interested in creating their own variations on these traditional forms. Many yoga teachers teach in eclectic styles, having been influenced by a number of methods. Hatha has proven to be a practice that continues to change and evolve with the times, while remaining true to the essential principles of the philosophy. Physical health and fitness level and personal goals will determine which style is best for the individual. The following list describes the styles most commonly practiced today.

Ananda: A gentle and meditative approach developed by Swami Kriyananda, this system places emphasis on deeply relaxing into the poses along with the use of **affirmations**, with the view that hatha's ultimate purpose is to heighten self-awareness.

Ashtanga: This is an intense and vigorous system developed by K. Pattabhi Jois and is characterized by equal emphasis on strength, flexibility, balance, and stamina. A modified version of this system is taught and often called "power yoga" (see page 42).

Bikram: Developed by Bikram Choudhury, this intense routine consists of 26 postures, including many standing one-legged balances, and begins and ends with a pranayama technique. The focus of this style is to detoxify the system and to warm up the muscles, allowing for maximum mastery of the poses. Therefore, teachers often use a humidifier and set the thermostat at 80°F (27°C) or higher for this practice.

Integral: This system was developed by Swami Satchidananda and reflects the teachings of Swami Sivananda. This method promotes the integration of yoga principles into lifestyle and thought, with the advice to be "easeful, peaceful, and useful."

Iyengar: A precise and detailed system developed by B.K.S. Iyengar, this style emphasizes correct postural alignment and proper body mechanics. The use of props and therapeutic applications are also characteristic of this style.

Kripalu: An internally directed approach developed by Yogi Amrit Desai, Kripalu is characterized by focusing on the breath and monitoring of the physical, mental, and emotional effects of the practice. Intensity ranges from gentle to vigorous.

Kundalini: A moderate to intense practice developed by Yogi Bhajan, this style focuses on the activation of the **kundalini** (serpent power) energy, believed to be stored at the base of the spine. Many breathing techniques are employed, along with poses and meditation, to facilitate the release of this energy.

Sivananda: This is a five-point method of practice that includes proper exercise, breathing, deep relaxation, vegetarian diet, and positive thinking through meditation. Swami Sivananda's system was popularized by Swami Vishnu-devananda and follows a standard format that includes breathing techniques, Sun Salutations, 12 yoga postures, relaxation, and chanting and prayers at the beginning and end of each class.

Viniyoga: Developed by T.K.V. Desikachar, this style employs a step-by-step approach (**vinyasa krama**) and emphasizes the use of the breath during **asana** practice. Another characteristic of this technique is the focus on tailoring the practice to the individual. Teachers of this system often design therapeutic applications.

Chapter Two

Teaching a Yoga Class

Equipment

Yoga practice requires few props and no special attire. However, the following suggestions support a safe and beneficial workout.

Props

There are many accessible items that are useful. Bare walls, folding chairs, platforms, and benches are great when adaptations are indicated. Other commonly used pieces of equipment and yoga props include:

- **Blankets** Firmly woven blankets can be folded to support seated poses or rolled to cushion the joints in various positions and are also used for warmth when practicing breathing, relaxation, and meditation techniques.
- **Blocks** These are usually made of wood or a synthetic material and also have many uses, especially in assisting those with flexibility and balance challenges.

- **Bolsters** Bolsters are similar to sofa cushions, but are rounder and firmer. These are often used to make seated and supine poses more comfortable.
- **Chairs** The best chairs to use when practicing yoga are wood or metal, with a straight back and no arms. Chairs have many uses, but are especially helpful when modifying poses for participants who cannot get down to the floor.
- **Mirrors** While not mandatory and rarely found in traditional yoga schools, mirrors are quite useful for viewing alignment and form.
- **Stretching straps** There are two types of stretching straps: heavy cotton straps with buckles and thick elastic resistance bands. They have many uses, but are primarily used to stretch the hamstrings.
- **Yoga mats** These mats are made of a rubber-like material and provide traction for standing poses and padding for floor-work (i.e., seated, prone, and supine positions). They are often called sticky mats because they stick to hard or smooth surfaces.

Attire

While no specific clothing is required for yoga, it is recommended that outfits are comfortable and that the feet are bare. Tights and leotards or shorts and T-shirts are appropriate. Attire should be non-restrictive, but not too baggy. The body's form should be visible so that the alignment of the postures is easily seen.

Environment

Yoga is taught in many different settings. It is not always possible to have an "ideal" environment: wood floor, bare walls, adjustable lighting and temperature, yoga props, and a soundproof room. Teachers need to be flexible and work with what is available. Make sure that unnecessary equipment and furniture are moved out of the way and place participants so that they have enough space to move safely.

Each individual should have enough space to stand with legs spread and arms stretched out to the side. Participants should also be able to lie on the floor with legs straight, arms stretched out to the side, or arms stretched overhead on the floor.

Yoga should be practiced in a clean, uncluttered environment with ample air circulation. The floor surface should be firm, preferably wood, or a no-nap or industrial carpet. A yoga sticky mat is the most important piece of equipment.

Music

Although chanting is an integral part of many traditional hatha practices (i.e., Sivananda, Integral, Kundalini), music is not. However, music can promote a relaxed atmosphere and many teachers use it. New Age music, which is instrumental and nondescript, seems to work best. The volume should be low and never override verbal cues. The pace should be slow and devoid of pronounced rhythm as well.

Personal Limitations

Pay attention to the health considerations and fitness levels of your participants. Be well versed in the safety guidelines and considerations, and request a health profile including past history of injury or surgery, and any other health considerations, such as carpal tunnel syndrome, arthritis, or pregnancy. Are they taking any medication? At the very least, make a verbal inquiry at the beginning of each class: How is everybody doing today? Does anyone have a special concern?

Ideally, yoga classes should be both classified and qualified. For example:

Power Yoga: Beginners' prep class

Power Yoga: Intense and vigorous, for those athletically inclined

Gentle Yoga: All levels welcome

Gentle Yoga: Soft and mellow, for those in need of relaxation and stress reduction

This will help regulate class participation and prevent injury.

Modifications

Most postures can be modified or adapted to an individual's needs by breaking the pose down into parts and teaching it in stages, starting on a basic level and building from there. For instance, you should teach the feet and leg positions and movements of a standing pose first, followed by the torso, arms, and head, ultimately putting all the pieces together. Use props for support and balance as needed, or for participants whose flexibility and/or weakness warrants an adaptation of the pose. (Teachers are advised to undergo training in prop usage before using them in yoga classes.)

Exercise Leadership

As a teacher you have many responsibilities. You share information and direct the participants through a lesson plan. You also monitor their efforts while being aware of safety considerations. Additionally, your delivery and guidance should be designed for maximum benefit and enjoyment. This section addresses the teaching skills necessary for effective instruction.

Verbal Introduction

Greet the class by welcoming them and introducing yourself. Give a brief description of your fitness background and yoga training. Describe the class program and its style, level, and content.

Risk Assessment / Health Screening

Get to know your participants' names and any pertinent physical issues concerning each. Remind them to listen to their bodies, not to force or strain, and to go at their own pace.

> **Query them as follows:**
> - Is there anyone new to this class today?
> - Have you ever done yoga before?
> - If so, what kind and how long have you been doing it?
> - Do you have any past injuries that I should know about?
> - How's everyone doing today?
> - Is there anything going on (physically) with any of you?

Technique Review

Before you begin the class, remind participants of the following:
- Body placement will be directed first; remember the importance of alignment.
- Breathe consciously and rhythmically; coordinate breath and movement.
- Do not force or strain; seek to be steady and comfortable at all times.

As in all group fitness instruction, proper cueing is vital. In yoga, you need to direct body placement and breathing patterns, as well as convey the purpose of the pose or breathing technique. Voice quality and demeanor are also important. A clear, well-modulated voice delivered in a gentle but commanding manner is desirable. The following represents general teaching technique and cueing format.

- Name the pose, describing its components, purpose, and benefits.
- Demonstrate the pose.
- Guide basic placement of the beginning position, including major parts of the body: feet, legs, torso, arms, and head.
- Direct breathing to be conscious, slow, and even.
- Cue movements into the pose, indicating coordination of breath and movement.
- Remind participants to breathe rhythmically as the pose is held.
- Continually direct attention to key points of placement and body awareness, including cautionary notes on alignment and mechanics.
- Remind participants to listen to their bodies and give them permission to come out of the pose earlier than directed, if needed.
- Verbally guide participants out of the pose, encouraging them to keep their awareness of the body and their breath.
- Return to the starting position and encourage participants to remain still for several breaths while they focus on their experience of the posture.

Chapter Three

Basic Asana Repertoire

Standing Poses

Tadasana (Mountain Pose)

Stand tall but relaxed with your feet firmly planted on the ground, together or hip-width apart. Keep your shoulders down and your abdomen pulled in and up. Arms are at your sides, palms turned toward your legs. Visualize a vertical line connecting your earlobe, shoulder, and the sides of the hip, knee, and ankle. Look straight ahead.

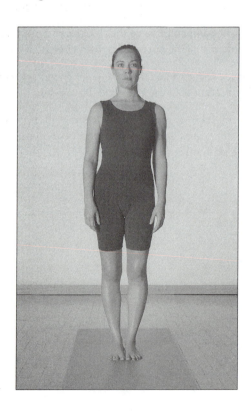

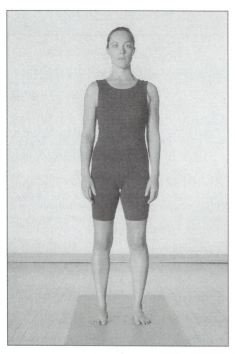

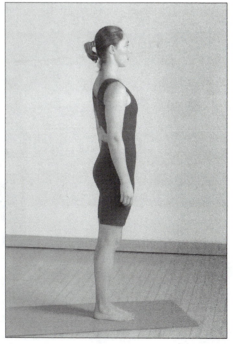

FITNESS YOGA

15

Standing Poses *(continued)*

Utkatasana (Chair Pose)

Begin in Mountain Pose. Separate your feet hip-width. Inhale as you bring your arms up in front of you to shoulder height, keeping them shoulder-distance apart with the palms facing the floor. Exhale as you bend your knees, releasing your buttocks back and down as though you are going to sit in a chair. Keep your heels flat on the floor, your shoulders down, and chest lifted. Make sure that your knees track in line with your hips and feet. Keep your weight pressing backwards. Look forward. Inhale as you come up out of the pose. Note: Modification using wall as prop.

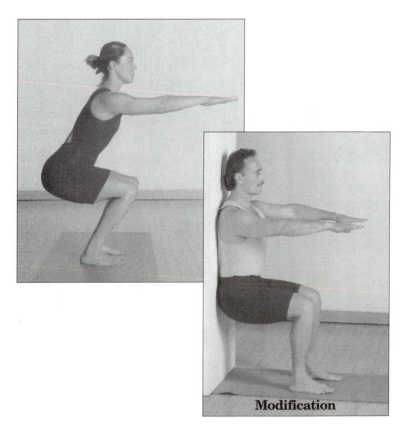

Modification

Standing Poses (continued)

Utthita Trikonasana (Triangle Pose)

Begin in Mountain Pose. Separate your legs to about 3½ to 4 feet apart. Turn your right foot out 90 degrees and your left foot in 30 degrees. The right heel should be in line with the arch of the left foot. Inhale and raise your arms to the sides at shoulder height. Exhale as you reach out and down over the right leg. Place your hand on your shin or on the floor behind the right foot. Your left arm is reaching straight up on a vertical line. Turn your head and look up at the left hand. Repeat to the other side. Note: Modification using a block.

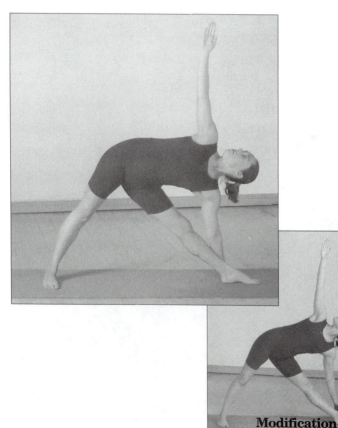

Modification

Standing Poses *(continued)*

Uttanasana (Forward Bend Pose)

Begin in Mountain Pose. Place your hands on your hips and inhale. Exhale as you bend forward, pivoting at the hips. Keep your quadriceps contracted, lifting your kneecaps. Place your hands outside your feet and bring your head toward your knees. Breathe deeply and keep your eyes open. Come up out of the pose slowly. Note: Modifications using the wall and blocks as props.

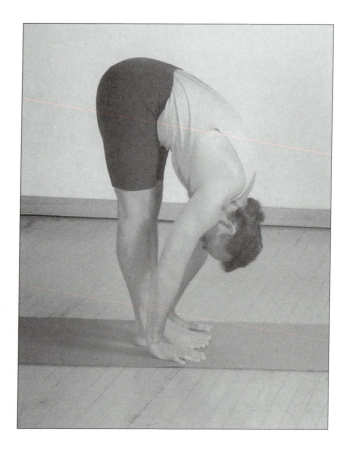

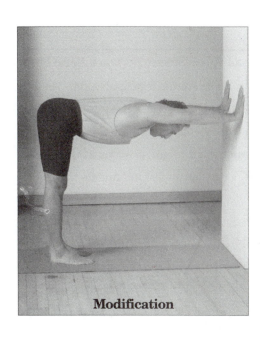

Modification

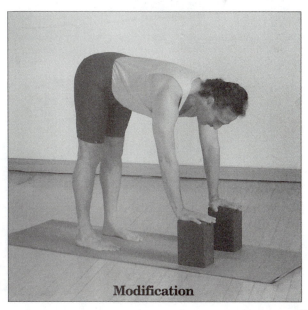

Modification

Standing Poses (continued)

Prasarita Padottanasana I (Wide Stance Forward Bend Pose)

Begin in Mountain Pose. Separate the legs to about $4^{1}/_{2}$ to 5 feet apart. Keep the feet facing forward with the toes slightly turned in. Place your hands at your hips and inhale. Lead with the chest as you exhale and bend forward, pivoting at the hips. Take hold of your big toes with your index and middle fingers. Draw your torso downward using the strength of your arms, bringing the top of the head to the floor. Keep your legs strong with the thighs contracted and kneecaps pulled up. To come out, place your hands or fingertips on the floor first. Then place your hands on your hips as you inhale. Pause and exhale. Then inhale and come up slowly. Note: Modification with blocks as props.

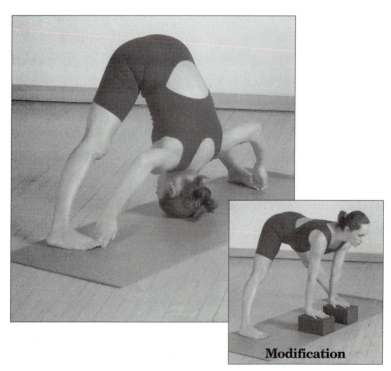

Modification

Standing Poses (continued)

Utthita Parsvakonasana (Side Angle Pose)

Begin in Mountain Pose. Separate the legs to about $4^{1}/_{2}$ to 5 feet apart. Turn your right foot out 90 degrees and your left foot in 30 degrees. Inhale and raise your arms up to the sides at shoulder level. Exhale and bend the right knee. The right leg should form a right angle with the thigh parallel to the floor and the shin perpendicular to the thigh. Reach to the right with the torso and place your right arm behind the right leg with the hand on the floor. Rotate your left arm open and bring it over your head. Turn your face and look toward the extended left hand. Inhale to come out and repeat to the other side. Note: Modified pose with arm placed on thigh and upper arm remaining in vertical alignment.

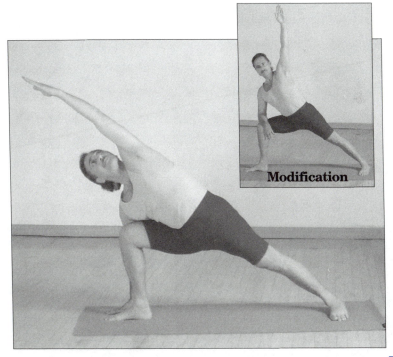
Modification

FITNESS YOGA

Balancing Posture

Vrksasana (Tree Pose)

Begin in Mountain Pose. Place the sole of your right foot on the inside of the upper left thigh. Open your right knee to the right. Keep your hips square and contract the thigh muscles of the standing leg. Bring your palms together at your heart center. Arms may also be stretched up overhead with the fingers interlaced, keeping the index fingers pointing up in "Steeple Mudra." Repeat on the other side.

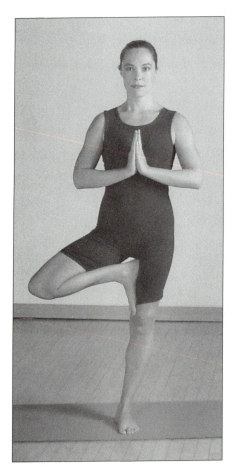
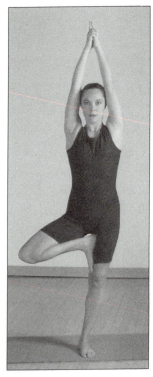

Seated Poses

Sukhasana (Easy Pose)

Sit on the floor and cross your legs at the ankles. Toes should be forward from the hips. Rest your arms on your legs with the palms up or down. Lengthen the spine by stretching your back in an upward motion and balance your head over the torso. Bring the chin down slightly so that the back of the neck is long, keeping the throat soft. Alternate the crossing of the legs with each practice. Note: Modification with folded blanket as prop.

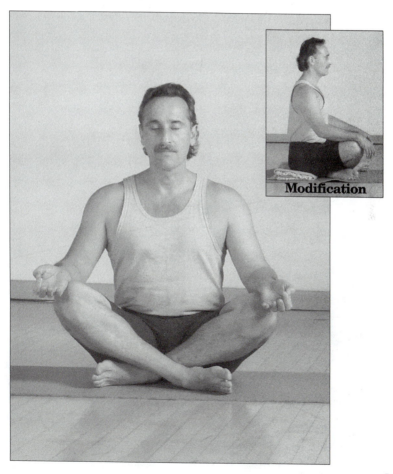
Modification

Seated Poses (continued)

Dandasana (Staff Pose)

Sit with your legs stretched straight in front of you. Lift up from the hips so that the spine is straight. Extend through the legs, contracting the thighs and flexing the feet. Place the palms on the floor so that the fingertips are facing forward and in line with the hips. Engage your back muscles by drawing your shoulder blades downward. Lift your chest up and look down toward your heart. Note: Modification with blanket and strap as props.

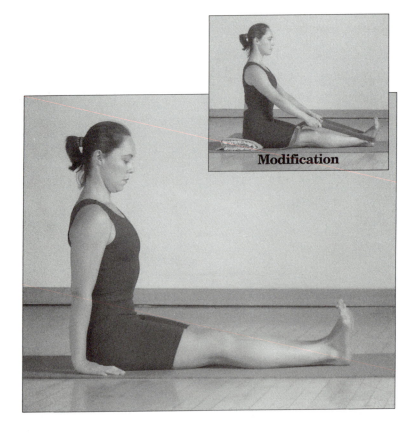

Modification

Seated Poses *(continued)*

Janusirsasana (Head-to-knee Pose)

Begin in Staff Pose. Bend the left knee to the side, bringing the sole of the left foot on the inside of the right upper thigh. Lean forward, pivoting at the hips and leading with the chest. Interlace your fingers around the ball of the right foot. Inhale and lift your torso up and over the thigh. Exhale as you stretch your head toward your knee. Keep the right leg active by extending through the back of the leg, contracting your quadriceps, and pressing through the heel. Keep the foot active by drawing the toes toward you. Breathe deeply and inhale when you come out of the pose. Repeat on the other side. Note: Modification with blanket and strap as props.

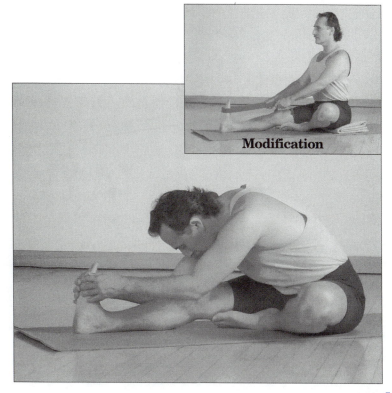

Seated Poses (continued)

Chatushpada Pitham (Table Pose)

Begin in Staff Pose. Bend your knees and place your feet hip-distance apart, toes pointing forward. Keep your arms shoulder-width apart or wider and bring your hands behind the line of your hips, approximately 6 to 8 inches, with the fingers pointing forward. Inhale and bend your elbows slightly. Exhale and roll your tailbone up from the floor, lifting your hips and back to a horizontal alignment. Let your head release back. The arms and shins should be perpendicular to the floor. Note: Modify this pose by keeping the head forward. If wrists are sensitive, turn the fingers away from hips.

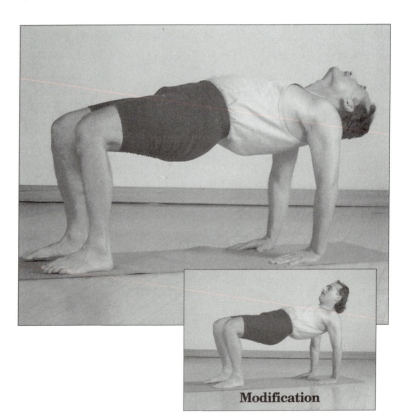

Modification

Seated Poses (continued)

Marichyasana III (Seated Twist)

Begin in Staff Pose. *Stage One/Beginners*: Use a folded blanket to support your hips. Bend the left knee, placing the foot in toward the left hip. The left shin should be perpendicular to the floor. Bring your left arm behind your left buttock or hip with the palm flat on the floor. Stretch your right arm up, lengthening your torso and, as you twist toward the left, bend your right elbow bringing it to the outside of your thigh or knee. Keep your shoulders even and your head centered. Repeat to the other side.

Stage Two/Advanced: Follow directions for Stage One, deleting the blanket as prop. Complete the pose by wrapping the arms around the back and clasping the hands or either wrist. The head may be turned either to look over the shoulder or toward the extended foot. Repeat to the other side.

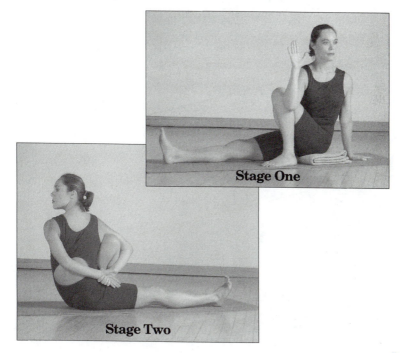

Prone Poses

Chakravakasana (Cat Stretch Pose)

On your hands and knees, place your hands underneath your shoulders and your knees underneath your hips, hip-distance apart. Begin with a neutral spine and look at the floor. Inhale and look up, arching the back. Exhale and look down, rounding the back. Repeat several times.

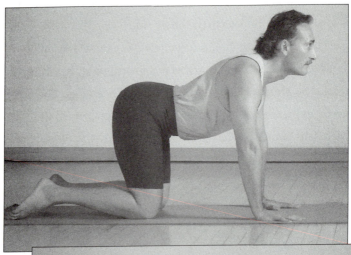

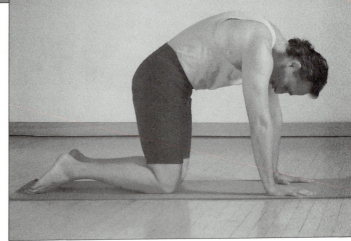

Prone Poses (continued)

Salabhasana (Locust)

Lie on your stomach with your legs hip-width apart and the tops of the feet on the floor. *Stage One/Beginners*: Bring your arms to your sides near your hips with the palms facing up. Inhale the breath and, as you exhale, raise your arms, chest, neck, and head. Keep your feet on the floor and look at the floor with the neck in neutral alignment. Hold and breathe. Exhale as you lower down.

Stage Two/Advanced: Bring your legs together and your arms out to the sides at shoulder level with the palms facing the floor. Inhale as your lift the arms, legs, chest, neck, and head up from the floor. Look forward and pull your arms back and up. Keep the legs together. Hold and breathe. Exhale as you lower down.

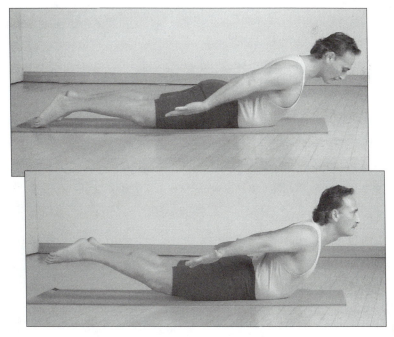

Supine Poses

Apanasana (Knee-to-chest Pose with Twist)

Lie on your back with your knees bent and feet on the floor at hip-width. *Stage One*: Inhale, and as you exhale bend your right knee and bring it up toward your chest. Clasp the hands underneath the knee or on top of the shin. Keep the head on the floor and the shoulders relaxed. Extend the left leg straight, flexing that foot. Hold and breathe for several breaths. *Stage Two*: Bring your right arm to the side at shoulder level with the palm up or down. Inhale and place your left hand over the right knee. As you exhale, bring the right knee over toward the left. Keep your right shoulder on the floor and look toward the right. Exhale as you recover center and repeat Stages One and Two to the left side.

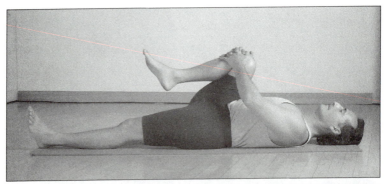

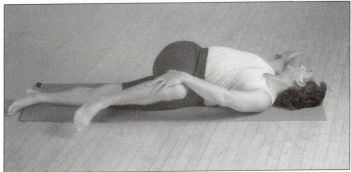

Supine Poses (continued)

Dvipada Pitham (Platform Pose)

Lie on your back and bend your knees, placing your feet hip-width apart. Heels should be away from the buttocks so that the shins remain perpendicular to the floor. Place your arms at your sides near the hips, with the palms flat on the floor. Inhale to prepare, and as you exhale roll your hips up from the floor. Maintain a "pelvic tilt" with the tailbone pointing upwards. Lengthen the spine and keep the ribs and throat soft with the neck extended. Do not grip the buttocks or try to arch the spine. Hold up and breathe. Exhale as you lower down.

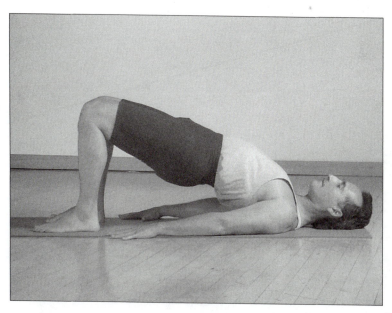

Supine Poses *(continued)*

Supta Padangusthasana (Supine Leg Stretch)

Lie on the floor with legs straight. *Stage One/Beginners*: Use a strap for this variation. Bend your right leg and place the strap around the bottom of the foot with an end in each hand. Inhale the breath, and as you exhale slowly straighten the right leg. Keep your shoulders relaxed, the neck long and the head centered. Hold and breathe for several breaths. Repeat to the other side. *Stages Two and Three/Advanced*: Begin as you did for Stage One without using the strap. Inhale and bend your right

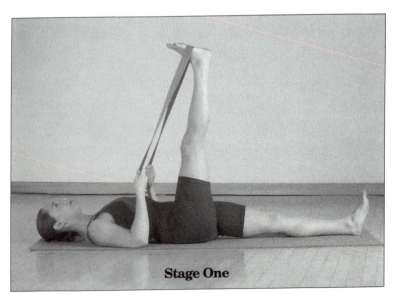

Stage One

leg and take hold of the big toe with your right index and middle fingers. Your left arm is stretched out to the left at shoulder level with the palm up or down. As you exhale, straighten the right leg. Your left leg is straight with the foot flexed. Inhale, and as you exhale rotate the leg out and bring it to the right. Keep your left buttock in contact with the floor. Turn your head and look toward the left. Exhale as you bring the leg back to center. Inhale and place your left hand on the left thigh. Exhale as you curl your torso, bringing your head toward your knee and your knee toward your head. Breathe deeply as you hold, and reach your left hand toward your left knee. Inhale as you come out of the pose. Repeat to the other side.

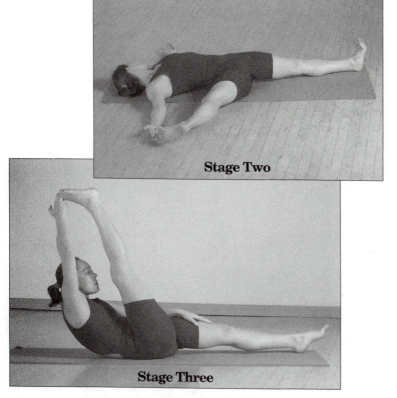

Inverted Pose

Viparita Karani Mudra

Lie on your back with your knees bent and feet flat on the floor at hip width. Rest your arms along the sides of the body, palms down. Exhale and push the palms down, draw the bent knees in and up, and straighten your legs as you lift your hips. Raise the hips to a comfortable angle of 45 to 75 degrees. Bend your elbows and bring your hands to the back of your pelvis and then slide the hands up to the lower back. Be sure that your legs are straight but not locked. The legs remain at an angle with the feet directly above your head.

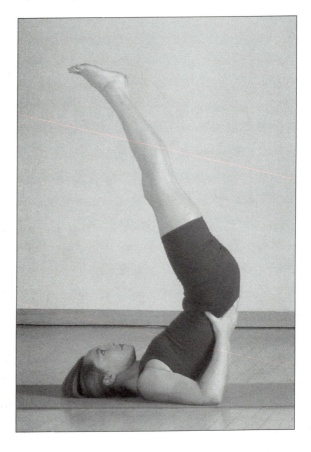

Sun Salutation

Surya Namaskar

A. Basic Stance (Tadasana)

Begin in Mountain Pose with your hands in prayer position at your heart.

B. Back Bend

Inhale and stretch your arms up as you arch back. Keep your buttocks and legs firm.

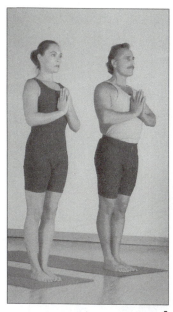

A.

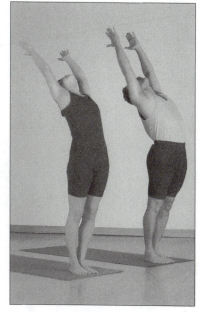

B.

Sun Salutation (continued)

Surya Namaskar

C. Forward Bend (Uttanasana)

Exhale and stretch forward and down from the hips. Place your hands in line with your toes, palms flat if possible. Draw your head toward your knees.

D. Lunge

Inhaling, reach your right leg straight back. The left foot remains in between the hands. Lift your head and chest and look forward. Retain the breath.

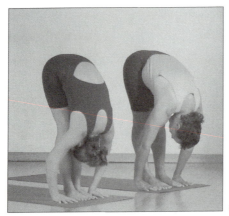

C.

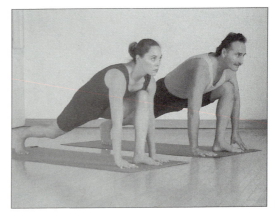

D.

Sun Salutation (continued)

Surya Namaskar

E. Plank Position

Reach your left leg back to meet the right. Keep back and legs straight and abdominal muscles firm. Look at the floor, with the head in line with the spine.

F. Pose of Eight Points

Exhale, bending your elbows and lowering your knees, chest, and chin to the floor. Arch your back and lift your buttocks in preparation for the Cobra Pose.

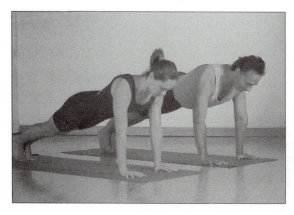

E.

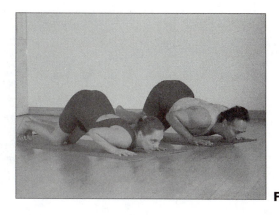

F.

Sun Salutation *(continued)*

Surya Namaskar

G. Cobra (Bhujangasana)

Inhale, lower your hips, point your toes, and lift your chest. Straighten your arms and look up, keeping the legs, hips, and feet on the floor. Press shoulders down in the opposite direction of the earlobes and keep the buttocks firm.

H. Downward-facing Dog (Adho Mukha Svanasana)

Curl your toes under and, exhaling, press up and back to an inverted V position. Keep neck relaxed and in between the arms. Lengthen the spine, keep your thighs firm, straighten the knees, and press the heels down.

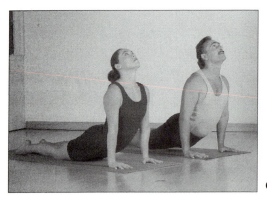

G.

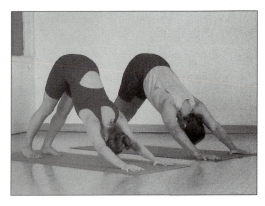

H.

Sun Salutation (continued)

Surya Namaskar

I. Lunge

Lift your head, inhale, and bring your right foot forward between your hands.

J. Forward Bend (Uttanasana)

Exhale and press from the ball of the left foot as you bring the left leg forward to meet your right leg. Straighten the knees, placing your hands on the outside of your feet, and bring your head toward your knees.

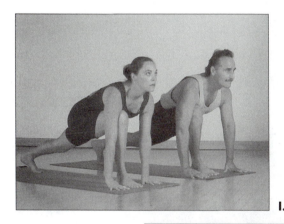

I.

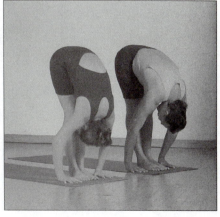

J.

Sun Salutation (continued)

Surya Namaskar

K. Arching Back

Inhale and lift with a straight back, arms alongside the head and neck. Knees stay straight, stomach firm. Look up and arch the back.

L. Basic Stance (Tadasana)

Exhaling, return to Mountain Pose, hands at chest in prayer position. Repeat the entire sequence, beginning with the left leg.

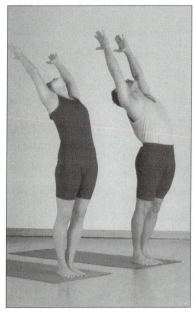

K.

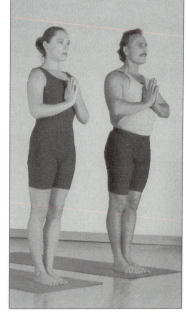

L.

Supine Pose

Savasana (Corpse or Relaxation Pose)

Lie flat on your back with your arms relaxed along the sides of your torso, palms up. Stretch the arms and legs and then relax them. Keep the arms slightly away from the trunk, with the palms facing up. Allow the legs and feet to roll away from each other. Place a folded towel under the head, a bolster under the knees, and a silk bag over the eyes to aid in your relaxation. Feel the weight of your body sinking into the floor and the mind becoming still. Breathe naturally and hold for three to 10 minutes.

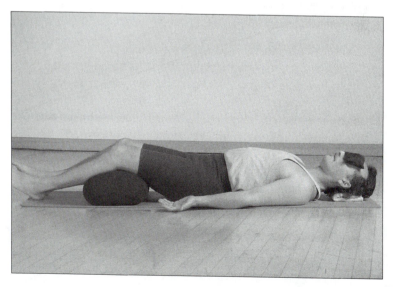

Power Yoga

Power yoga is a term used to describe a yoga class that is intense and vigorous. Originally used to describe an Ashtanga-style yoga class, this term is now used more loosely. Any yoga class that is a modification of an Ashtanga class or includes demanding poses and an intermittent flow of movement might be identified as a "power yoga" class. These classes are designed to create a balance of strength, flexibility, and stamina.

Cardiovascular Complication Risk and Screening
The characteristics of a power yoga class make it similar to interval training. When Sun Salutations are included they are usually repeated several times as a warm-up, then repeated throughout the class. Various poses are held for several breaths in between these repetitions. Accordingly, this type of class presents a higher cardiovascular risk and, therefore, should not be taught to participants who have existing cardiovascular or valvular disease, hypertension, non-insulin-dependent diabetes, or who are significantly overweight. Participants should be physically fit; therefore cardiovascular screening is recommended.

Strength Benefits and Injury Risk
There are tremendous strength benefits to be gained from this type of yoga workout. Power yoga classes include many postures that develop strength in the legs, back, and abdominals as well as weightbearing poses that build upper-body strength. A frequently performed upper-body pose in a power yoga class is the yoga-style push up, Chaturanga Dandasana. This posture and other postures that entail arm balancing of some sort present a risk to the wrists, elbows, and shoulders.

Cautionary Notes
Teaching this type of class involves added responsibility

because of its intensity and the accompanying safety issues. You should be experienced and trained in the more vigorous styles of yoga before teaching in this fashion. Newcomers to yoga will benefit from taking a beginner's yoga course to become familiar with a basic repertoire of asanas and studying for several months before joining a power yoga class. Therefore, it is wise to screen your participants. In power yoga, proper alignment and good body mechanics are crucial. A preparatory class in which the poses and sequences are broken down is recommended. People with back problems or joint issues should approach this style cautiously. Power yoga is not recommended for people with hypertension or heart problems.

Chapter Four

Breath Awareness

Breath Awareness Techniques (Pranayama)

Abdominal Breathing

Synonymous with deep diaphragmatic breathing and often called the "belly breath," abdominal breathing is recommended as a way to focus attention, calm the mind, and increase oxygen intake. Breathe in through the nose and out through the nose or mouth. Draw the breath into the abdomen, expanding to the front, back, and sides. On the exhalation, contract the abdominal area.

Chest Breathing

During chest breathing, the focus is on the inhalation and on the chest area as the breath is drawn in. This is recommended as a way to energize and improve poor posture. Expand equally from the center of the chest in all directions. Let the chest soften on the exhalation. Breathe in through the nose and out through the nose or mouth.

Lengthening the Breath

In general, yoga directs us to slow down our breathing, making the breaths long and slow, with the inhalations and exhalations equal in length. The next step is to make the breaths uneven. Making the exhalation longer than the inhalation promotes a deeper state of calm; lengthening the inhalation energizes the mind and the body.

Breath Retentions

Breath retentions involve retaining or holding the breath at the end of an inhalation. Initially, this should only be a pause of two to five seconds.

Breath Suspensions

The opposite of a retention, breath suspension is the holding of the breath out at the end of the exhalation. Again, this should only last two to five seconds.

Breath with Sound (Ujjayi)

Breathing with sound involves making a sound on both the inhalation and exhalation by constricting the throat and breathing in and out through the nose. The sound is soft and resembles ocean waves at a distance.

Note: Almost all traditional yoga breathing techniques prescribe both inhaling and exhaling through the nose.

Chapter Five

Programming

The word yoga means union. Hatha is often translated as Ha signifying the sun, and Tha, the moon. Hatha also means force, power, and effort. Every aspect of the technique is based on the principle of the union of opposites. Thus, hatha yoga is a very powerful system that facilitates a harmonious psychophysiological state of being. The repertoire of hatha includes poses, or asanas, and breathing techniques collectively called pranayama.

Asana literally means seat, posture, or pose. Spinal health is an important factor. The structure of a yoga class consists of poses that take the spine through its full range of motion: forward, backward, lateral, and rotated. Postures are performed while standing, seated, prone, and supine. Additionally, there are inverted poses such as the shoulder stand. A well-rounded asana practice can improve your posture, build strength, and promote greater flexibility at any age.

Pranayama means breath control or life force extension and affects the body energetically. The practice begins with conscious breath awareness exercises and ultimately includes very sophisticated techniques. Various breathing exercises can energize the body while others will relax and calm the system. The most important thing is to breathe slowly and consciously.

Poses and breathing practices include characteristics that are paired as follows: expansion and contraction, pose and counterpose, dynamic and static, steadiness and comfort. What this means is that each pose and breathing technique possesses dualistic qualities that are complementary. For instance, we expand as we inhale and contract as we exhale; when we perform a pose that requires extension of the spine, such as the cobra, we need to perform a counterpose that will bring the spine into flexion, such as a seated forward bend. Dynamic, in hatha, indicates movement and activity, while static is represented by holding and stillness. The Sun Salutation is a perfect example of moving dynamically with asana. The Breath of Fire (exhaling rapidly) is considered a dynamic breathing practice. In the Viniyoga system, the dynamic approach — moving into and out of a posture several times before holding — is frequently applied. The Iyengar system, in contrast, mostly dictates the static mode. All postures and breathing techniques should be performed with steadiness and comfort.

> Do not confuse dynamic with aggressive — you can gently move into and out of a pose. And static — being still — does not mean easy. Holding a standing pose for 60 seconds can be quite intense!

Frequency of Practice

Yoga is intended to be practiced every day, although this goal is difficult for most people to attain. For minimum benefit, a 90-minute class taken twice a week is recommended. Also, specific yoga poses can be substituted for the stretches that are routinely done after strength and cardiovascular workouts. Therefore, a mini routine of 10 to 15 minutes could easily be integrated into one's fitness regimen three to five times a week.

Dedicated practitioners whose main fitness activity is yoga routinely take a one- to two-hour class two or more times a week, supplemented by 20 to 30 minutes of daily home practice sessions.

Components

Class formatting guidelines for yoga are quite similar to those suggested for other group fitness activities. Be prepared with a lesson plan that fits into the alloted time and includes a warm-up sequence, the body of the class (including poses and counterposes), and time for relaxation. The warm-up should include stretches and poses that prepare the body for the workout. It is important to pace your delivery, allowing time for questions, discussion, and the possibility of special circumstances.

> Relaxation at the end of class is equivalent to, and as important as, the cooling down segment of generic fitness classes. It should never be rushed. Plan a five- to 10-minute relaxation for a 45-minute to one-hour class, and a 10- to 15-minute segment for classes of 75 minutes to two hours in length.

Safety Rules

Although yoga is often thought of as "kind and gentle" to the body, its practice requires as much caution as any other form of exercise. In addition to the general guidelines, class content is influenced by the fitness level and specific considerations of the participants. Obviously, a yoga workout designed for heart patients will be quite different from one intended for triathletes. participants must let their teachers know about any health concerns and past injuries or surgeries. Instructors must be trained to assess participants' capabilities and state of health. Never manually or verbally force a student into a pose. While physical touch may promote the refinement of posture and enhance movement, aggressive adjustments must be avoided.

Injury Prevention

Along with the popularity of yoga — especially power yoga — a growing liability concern has emerged. As with any fitness modality, instructors who teach yoga need to approach their work conscientiously, pairing the appropriate training with awareness and responsibility. Teach only what you know and be prepared for your specific student population. A 30- to 40-minute private evaluation session with new participants is recommended to determine the class style and level that is appropriate.

Contraindications/High-risk Poses

Specific poses and breathing techniques are believed to prevent or even remedy many physical and mental conditions. Similarly, there are poses and techniques that are contraindicated for specific health issues. The following are the most common:

Menstruation

During menstruation, women should not practice inverted postures such as hand, head, or shoulder stands. However, viparita karani, a modified shoulder stand, is acceptable if it is comfortable. A vigorous practice that includes backbends and numerous standing poses is also discouraged. Gentler practice is recommended at this time of the month. A restorative practice that focuses on forward bends and relaxation techniques will be more effective in combating the discomforts common at this time.

Pregnancy

Pregnant women should not perform inverted postures or extended breath retentions (holding the breath in after the inhalation) or suspensions (holding the breath out after the exhalation). Holding the breath in or out may limit blood flow to the fetus. Abdominal contractions such as the stomach lift are strictly forbidden. Essentially, pregnant women are given the same advice regarding yoga as they are in general fitness: Check with your physician before starting a new program and do not do anything drastically different from what you are accustomed to. Note that there are yoga teachers that specialize in prenatal yoga.

Sciatica

If sciatica is a concern, the participant should not perform poses that require extreme flexion and intense stretching of the hamstrings. These include most of the forward-bending poses. Conversely, medical doctors, physical therapists, and chiropractors often recommend back extensions with poses such as the cobra as a remedy for this condition.

Controversial Poses

There are several yoga poses that fall into the category of high-risk exercises. They are the shoulder stand, the plow, and the headstand, all of which are considered inversions in yoga. Many of the advanced back-bending poses that involve hyperextension of the spine are also suspect. With proper training and performed with correct body mechanics, all of these poses can be extremely beneficial and therapeutic. Practiced improperly, they can be dangerous and create serious liability concerns.

Shoulder Stand/Plow —The shoulder stand and plow both involve extreme flexion of the neck. Additionally, the plow requires substantial flexibility in the back muscles and hamstrings. Allowances can be made for the lack of flexibility by modifying the poses and the support of props. Viparita Karani (shown on page 34) can be considered a modified shoulder stand. This pose entails less flexion in the legs, back, and hamstrings and therefore does not require props. It is generally considered the safest of all the inverted postures.

Headstand —The headstand requires back and arm strength as well as abdominal strength. Neck problems preclude the practice of this pose entirely. The handstand, commonly practiced in the Ashtanga and Iyengar styles of yoga, requires the same strength as the headstand but is less problematic for the neck.

Backbends —Although previously considered risky or unsafe, the cobra posture is now routinely presented in fitness classes. This pose is similar to the McKenzie back extension exercise that is frequently prescribed by back specialists, chiropractors, and physical therapists. Leaders in both the medical and fitness industries agree that back extension is necessary to counteract the slouching posture promoted by so much chair sitting in today's culture.

The locust, modified bridge, and bow are additional back-bending poses that are beneficial and safe to practice. More advanced back-bending poses such as the wheel are more risky as they entail more action in the shoulders, elbows, and wrists.

Group yoga instructors should stick to the least risky of these postures. The modified shoulder stand (Viparita Karani) is the safest inverted posture, unless otherwise contraindicated (see Contraindications/High-risk Poses, page 49). The cobra and locust are your best bets for back-bending poses, followed by the bridge and the bow. The other poses discussed above should only be taught by very experienced yoga instructors and only when appropriate (i.e., in small classes with participants who are properly prepared and able.)

Hypertension, high blood pressure, glaucoma, eye problems, and ear congestion

Participants with these conditions should not practice breath retentions, inverted poses, or prolonged standing forward bends. A practice that is slow-paced, gentle, and promotes relaxation is appropriate for individuals with these conditions.

Intensity Monitoring

While a degree of deep feeling and intensity may accompany a yoga practice, participants should not be encouraged to push themselves beyond a reasonable degree of challenge. Using the breath to monitor effort and paying attention to how the body is responding are good ways to remain "steady and comfortable." Observe participants' breathing patterns and how they are holding a pose. When breathing is labored or erratic — or the body is shaking — the student is obviously working too hard. Teachers must closely observe participants and remind them to observe themselves so they can avoid such situations.

> Experienced yoga practitioners will use the breath and body awareness rather than the clock to gauge performance duration. For example, a seated forward bend might be held for 10 to 15 slow breaths and a back bend might be held for three to seven breaths. The practitioner completes the pose when it feels right to come out, the breaths are no longer smooth, and/or the maximum point of challenge has been met.

Most importantly, reiterate the following:
- Monitor the breath; it should be smooth and even, never labored.
- Feel the body; if there is pain, back off.

- Avoid poses that activate pain.
- Pace yourself; if you feel the need to rest, do so.

Be sensitive to participants' response to your lesson plan. If class content seems too advanced, lighten up the intensity by either doing more basic posture modifications or reducing the number of repetitions and the length of time each pose is held. Conversely, if your participants seem able to do more, you can keep the same lesson plan, but intensify it by increasing the number of repetitions and the length of holding the poses.

A general rule for a beginner is to repeat a pose three to five times, holding each repetition for a duration of five to 20 seconds. As participants become more skilled, postures can be repeated only once or twice, but held for greater lengths of time — 15 to 30 seconds. But this rule is further qualified by additional cri-

> **General Guidelines**
> The following points ensure a safe and effective yoga practice.
> - Do not eat right before class. Allow two to three hours after a 800 – 1200 calorie meal, one to two hours after lighter meals (250 – 800 calories), and 30 minutes to one hour after a snack (fewer than 250 calories).
> - Dress comfortably. Feet should be bare.
> - Practice on a non-skid surface.
> - Make sure you have enough room to move freely.
> - Space should be free of unnecessary equipment and furniture.
> - Room temperature should be neutral to warm with good air circulation. Cold temperatures are not conducive to flexibility.
> - Avoid practicing outside in direct sunlight in hot and humid climates, especially during the peak hours of sunshine (i.e., between 10 AM and 2 PM).
> - Focus on what you are doing and listen to your body. Do not force or strain.
> - Breathe slowly and rhythmically through the nose. Do not hold the breath.

teria. More active poses such as backbends and standing postures are generally held for shorter durations (60 seconds or less), while passive postures such as forward bends and seated poses can be held for longer lengths of time (60 seconds or more).

Sample Class

The following poses constitute a well-rounded yoga class. Remember to include warm-up and cool-down segments (See Components, page 48).

Standing Poses
Tadasana / Mountain Pose
Utkatasana / Chair Pose
Uttanasana / Forward Bend
Utthita Trikonasana / Triangle Pose
Prasarita Padottanasana I / Wide Stance Forward Bend
Vrksasana / Tree Pose

Prone Poses
Chakravakasana / Cat Stretch
Adho Mukha Svanasana / Downward-facing Dog Pose
Bhujangasana / Cobra Pose

Seated Poses
Sukhasana / Easy Pose
Janusirsasana / Head-to-knee Pose
Marichyasana III / Seated Twist

Supine Poses
Apanasana / Knee-to-chest Pose
Dvipada Pitham / Platform Pose
Savasana / Corpse or Relaxation Pose

Chapter Six

Yoga Teacher Standards and Certification

Becoming a yoga teacher involves more than learning poses. If you are already a trained fitness or health professional but are new to yoga, you may begin to incorporate what you learn about yoga into your teaching routine and even teach a "yoga-based stretch class," for instance. But you must continue your yoga training. Yoga is a sophisticated practice, much more than merely a unique piece of choreography. There are many facets to becoming a yoga teacher. In addition to learning body mechanics, including anatomy and physiology, and studying the poses and breathing techniques, you need to have a foundation in yoga philosophy.

There is a wide range of training and certification programs available that reflect the many styles and traditions in yoga. Additionally, many of these schools are represented in a non-profit, volunteer organization called Yoga Alliance. This group has been formed to uphold the integrity of yoga and establish national standards for yoga teachers.

Glossary

The technique of yoga is described in Sanskrit, India's ancient language. Though it is not necessary to study Sanskrit extensively in order to benefit from or even teach yoga, you need to know a basic definition of terms. Therefore, it is recommended that you acquire a working vocabulary of the techniques. Learning the Sanskrit terms will give you greater insight into the meaning of yoga.

Affirmation – Positive statement made in the present tense, usually of nine words or less. Stated audibly or silently, with feeling, and accompanied by an image or visualization. Example: "I have a strong and flexible spine."

Asana – Literally, "seat;" also, "attitude." Asanas are the poses or positions that form the structure of hatha yoga.

Ashtanga Yoga – Literally, "eight-limbed discipline." As described by Patanjali in his classic treatise, *The Yoga Sutras*, the path of yoga is divided into eight steps. They are moral observance, self-discipline, posture, life force control, sensory transcendence, concentration, meditation, and absorption or enlightenment. Note that ashtanga yoga also describes a style of hatha yoga.

Chakra – Literally, "wheel" or "circle." Located along the spine, these energy centers correlate with actual physical functions. Psychological qualities are attributed to them as well. Considered storage places for **prana**, they are activated by specific postures and breathing exercises. Chakras, along with the **nadis**, mentioned below, make up the internal highway for the flow of prana.

Guru – Teacher, guide. Literally, "destroyer of darkness;" one who illuminates.

Hatha Yoga – The physical aspect of yoga. Commonly translated with "Ha" as Sun and "Tha" as moon. Hatha literally means forceful or powerful.

Karma – Literally, "action" or "cause and effect." Implied meaning is that your good works and service will result in good coming back to you, in this life and the next. Similarly, what we experience now is a result of past actions.

Kundalini – Literally, "she who is coiled" or "serpent power." Energy believed to be stored at the base of the spine that is stimulated by yoga techniques.

Mantra – A sound, phrase, or affirmation. Translated literally as "an instrument of thought." Mantras are used both silently and audibly (as in chanting) as a way to keep the mind focused prior to meditation.

Meditation – Uninterrupted concentration, or concentration that is inwardly directed to discover Truth or the Absolute.

Mind-Body Connection – (Also Body-Mind.) A term now commonly used in both the health and fitness industries referring to the intricate connection between the body and the mind — how what we think affects our state of health and how we treat our bodies affects the functioning of the mind.

Mudra – Literally, "seal." Specific hand positions and some asanas are called mudras because they lock or seal energy in the body for a particular purpose.

Nadis – A tubular organ of the subtle or unseen body through which energy flows. It correlates with the concept of the meridian pathways as used in the science of acupuncture.

Nirvana – State of absolute bliss. Literally, extinction (of individual existence) and emergence into cosmic awareness.

Om – Also aum. Like the Latin word omne, the Sanskrit word aum means "all" or "cosmic vibration," and conveys the concepts of omniscience, omnipresence, and omnipotence. Om is often chanted at the beginning and end of traditional yoga classes.

Prana – Literally, "life force." Pranayama, or breathing techniques, facilitate the way this life force is extended or refined. Pranayama is also an integral part of hatha yoga training.

Pundit – A Brahmanic scholar. Commonly, a learned or wise person.

Sthira and Sukha – Sthira means to be alert, steady, and firm. Sukha means joy, pleasure, and ease. These two qualities — steadiness and comfort — are essential in the practice of hatha yoga.

Swami – Literally, "owner" or "lord." Common title of respect for a spiritual person. A person who is master of himself or herself rather than of other people. Often used interchangeably with the word guru.

Vinyasa Krama – Sequencing within an asana and pranayama practice. The step-by-step process of structuring a yoga practice to create a specific result.

Yoga – Literally, "to yolk back;" also means union or discipline. Yoga techniques are designed to create physical health and mental well-being, ultimately promoting spiritual enlightenment.

Index

A

abdominal breathing, 44
absorption (enlightenment), 56
acupuncture, 57
Adho Mukha Svanasana
 (Downward-facing Dog), 38
affirmations, 5, 56
alignment, 12, 43
Ananda, 5
Apanasana (Knee-to-chest Pose
 with Twist), 30
arching back, 40
arm balancing, 42
arthritis, 10
Asana, 7, 43, 56
 defined, 46
 repertoire, 14–43
Ashtanga, 5, 42, 51
attire, 9, 53
aum (om), 58

B

backbends, 35, 51
back extensions, 50
balance, 5
balancing posture, 22
"belly breath," 44
Benson, Herbert, 4
Bhajan, Yogi, 6
Bhujangasana
 (Cobra), 38, 47, 50, 51
Bikram, 5–6
biofeedback, 4
blankets, 8
blocks, 8, 17, 18, 20
blood pressure, 52
body awareness, 52
body mechanics, 6
body-mind connection, 57
bolster, 9, 41
bow, 51
breath awareness techniques
 (Pranayama), 44–45
breathing, 13, 52, 53
 chest and abdominal, 44
 techniques, 4, 6, 46, 47
breath lengthening, 44–45
Breath of Fire, 47
breath retention, 45, 50
breath suspension, 45, 50
Breath with Sound (Ujjayi), 45
bridge, 51

C

cardiovascular screening, 42
carpal tunnel syndrome, 10
certification, 55
Chair Pose (Utkatasana), 16
chairs, 9
Chakra, 56
Chakravakasana
 (Cat Stretch Pose), 28–29
chanting, 6, 10, 57, 58
Chaturanga Dandasana, 42
Chatushpada Pitham
 (Table Pose), 26
chest breathing, 44

Choudhury, Bikram, 5
class outline, 54
clothing, 9, 53
Cobra
    (Bhujangasana), 38, 47, 50, 51
comfort, 47, 58
components, of yoga
    programming, 48
concentration, 56
contraindications, 49–50
Corpse, or Relaxation, Pose
    (Savasana), 41
cueing, 13, 14

D

Dandasana (Staff Pose), 24
Desai, Yogi Amrit, 6
Desikachar, T. K. V., 7
detoxification, 6
diabetes, 42
diaphragmatic breathing, 44
diet, 6
Downward-facing Dog
    (Adho Mukha Svanasana), 38
dualism, 47
duration, 52–54
Dvipada Pitham
    (Platform Pose), 31
dynamic and static, 47

E

ear congestion, 52
Easy Pose (Sukhasana), 23
eating, before class, 53
"eight-limbed discipline," 56
Emerson, Ralph Waldo, 3
enlightenment (absorption), 56
environment, 9–10
equipment, 8–9

evaluation session, 49
exercise leadership, 11–13
expansion and contraction, 47
eye problems, 52

F

flexibility, 5, 42, 46
Forward Bend
    (Uttanasana), 19–20, 36, 39, 50
frequency of practice, 48

G

gentle yoga, 11
glaucoma, 52
guidelines, for safety, 53
guru, 57, 58

H

hamstrings, 50
handstand, 51
Hatha yoga
    benefits, 4
    defined, 46, 57
    growth, 3–4
    history, 2–3
    styles, 5–7
headstand, 46, 51
Head-to-knee Pose
    (Janusirsasana), 25
health screening, 10, 12
high-risk procedures, 51
hypertension, 52

I

injury prevention, 49
Integral system, 6, 10

intensity monitoring, 52–54
inverted poses, 34, 46
Iyengar, B. K. S., 6
Iyengar, 6, 47, 51

J

Janusirsasana
   (Head-to-knee Pose), 25
Jois, K. Pattabhi, 5

K

Karma, 57
Kripalu, 6
Kriyananda, Swami, 5
Kundalini (Serpent Power)
   energy, 6
Kundalini system, 6, 10, 57

L

leadership, 11–13
lengthening the breath, 44–45
lesson plan, 48
life force. *see* Prana
life force control, 56
Locust (Salabhasana), 29, 51
lunge, 36, 39

M

Mantra, 57
Marichyasana III
   (Seated Twist), 27
mats, 9, 10
McKenzie back extension, 51
medications, 10
meditation, 4, 6, 56, 57
menstruation, 50

"mental stillness," 4
mind-body connection, 3, 57
mind-body exercise, 1, 4
mirrors, 9
modifications, 11, 53
Modified Bridge, 51
Modified Shoulder Stand
   (Viparita Karani), 51
moral observance, 56
Mountain Pose
   (Tadasana), 14–15, 35, 40
Mudra, 57
music, 10

N

Nadis, 56, 57
New Age music, 10
Nirvana, 58

O

om (aum), 58

P

pain, 52, 53
Patanjali, 2, 56
pelvic tilt, 31
plank position, 37
Platform Pose
   (Dvipada Pitham), 31
plow, 51
pose and counterpose, 47
Pose of Eight Points, 37
poses (Asanas), 5, 6, 46
   and breathing practices, 47
postural alignment, 6, 44, 46, 56
postures, yoga, 6
   modifications, 11
power yoga, 5, 11, 42–43, 49

Prana, 56, 58
Pranayama
 (Breath Awareness Techniques),
 6, 44–45, 46, 47, 58
Prasarita Padottanasana
 (Wide Stance Forward
 Bend Pose), 20
prayers, 6
pregnancy, 10, 50
programming, 46–54
prone poses, 28–29, 54
props, 8, 11
pundit, 58
push up, yoga-style, 42

R

relaxation, 6, 41, 48, 50
Relaxation, or Corpse, Pose
 (Savasana), 41
Relaxation Response, 4
risk assessment/
 health screening, 10, 12

S

safety guidelines, 10, 49
Salabhasana (Locust), 29
Sanskrit, 56
Satchidananda, Swami, 6
Savasana
 (Corpse, or Relaxation, Pose), 41
sciatica, 50
seated forward bend, 47
seated poses, 23–27, 54
Seated Twist
 (Marichyasana III), 27
self-awareness, 5
self-discipline, 56
sensory transcendence, 56
serpent power
 (Kundalini energy), 6

shaking, 52
shoulder stand, 46
shoulder stand/plow, 51
Side Angle Pose
 (Utthita Parsvakonasana), 21
silk eye bag, 41
Sivananda, 6, 10
Sivananda, Swami, 6
space, 53
spinal health, 46
Staff Pose (Dandasana), 24
stamina, 5, 42
standing poses, 14–21, 54
static mode, 47
steadiness and comfort, 47, 58
"Steeple Mudra," 22
Sthira, 58
sticky mat, 9, 10
stomach lift, 50
strength, 5, 42, 46
stretching straps, 9, 32
Sukha, 58
Sukhasana (Easy Pose), 23
sunlight, 53
Sun Salutation, 6, 35–40, 42, 47
supine poses, 30–33, 41, 54
Supta Padangusthasana
 (Supine Leg Stretch), 32–33
Surya Namaskar, 35–40
Swami, 58

T

Table Pose
 (Chatushpada Pitham), 26
Tadasana
 (Mountain Pose), 14–15, 35, 40
teacher standards, 55
technique review, 12–13
temperature, room, 53
therapeutic applications, 6, 7
Thoreau, Henry David, 3

training, of teachers, 55
Tree Pose (Vrksasana), 22
Triangle Pose
   (Utthita Trikonasana), 17

U

Ujjayi (Breath with
   Sound), 45
union, 46, 58
Utkatasana (Chair Pose), 16
Uttanasana
   (Forward Bend Pose), 19–20
Utthita Parsvakonasana
   (Side Angle Pose), 21
Utthita Trikonasana
   (Triangle Pose), 17

V

valvular disease, 42
vegetarian diet, 6
verbal introduction, 12
Viniyoga, 7, 47
Vinyasa Krama, 7, 58
Viparita Karani (Modified
   Shoulder Stand), 50, 51
Viparita Karani Mudra, 34
Vishu-devanada, Swami, 6
Vrksasana (Tree Pose), 22

W

warm-up sequence, 48
wheel, 51
Wide Stance Forward Bend Pose
   (Prasarita Padottanasana I), 20

Y

yoga. *see* Hatha yoga
Yoga Alliance, 55
yoga philosophy, 55
The Yoga Sutras (Patanjali),
   2, 56

References and Suggested Reading

Benson, H. (1976). *The Relaxation Response.* New York: Avon Books.

Birch, B.B. (1995). *Power Yoga: The Total Strength and Flexibility Workout.* New York: Simon and Schuster.

Carrico, M. and the editors of *Yoga Journal.* (1997). *Yoga Journal's Yoga Basics: The Essential Beginner's Guide to Yoga for a Lifetime of Health and Fitness.* New York: Henry Holt.

Couch, J. (1991). *The Runner's Yoga Book: A Balanced Approach to Fitness.* Berkeley, Cal.: Rodmell Press.

Desikachar, T.K.V. (1995). *The Heart of Yoga: Developing a Personal Practice.* Rochester, Vermont: Inner Traditions.

Feuerstein, G. (1997). *The Shambhala Encyclopedia of Yoga.* Boston, Mass.: Shambhala Publishers.

Feuerstein, G. & Payne, L. (1999). *Yoga for Dummies.* Foster City, Cal.: IDG Books.

Iyengar, B.K.S. (1966). *Light on Yoga.* New York: Schocken Books.

Mohan, A.G. (1995). *Yoga for Body, Breath and Mind: A Guide to Personal Reintegration.* Portland, Ore.: Rudra Press.

Pierce, M. & Pierce, M. (1996). *Yoga for Your Life: A Practice Manual of Breath and Movement for Every Body.* Portland, Ore.: Rudra Press.

Yoga Teacher Registry, *contact: Yoga Alliance, 234 S. Third Ave., West Reading, PA 19611; (877) YOGA-ALL (964-2255).*

Yoga Research and Education Center: *P.O. Box 1386, Lower Lake, CA 95457; (707) 928-9898; www.yrec.org; e-mail: mail@yrec.org*

NOTES

NOTES

NOTES

NOTES

ABOUT THE AUTHOR

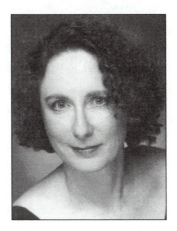

Known as the *Yoga Lady*,™ San Diego–based Mara Carrico is the author of *Yoga Journal's Yoga Basics* and a founding member of IDEA's Mind-Body Fitness Committee. Carrico is recognized as a Continuing Education Specialist for the American Council on Exercise and conducts Yoga for the West™ Teacher Training courses under the aegis of *YogaLink*™ International.

SPONSOR

YOGAFIT TRAINING SYSTEMS WORLDWIDE delivers nationally approved CEC/CEU programs for fitness instructors who wish to teach yoga in the fitness/health club environment. YogaFit is a user-friendly, fitness style of yoga specifically designed for fitness/health club members and staff.

Teaching yoga in a fitness facility has many challenges, including:
- Noisy distractions
- Bright lighting
- Cold group-exercise rooms
- Lack of equipment
- Multi-level participants in every class

YogaFit teaches fitness professionals to instruct a safe and very effective yoga class. YogaFit delivers an incredible body/mind workout in as little as 55 minutes and has trained thousands of fitness professionals and body workers around the world.

For more information go to www.yogafit.com or call (310) 376-1036.

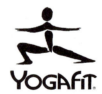

To locate this or any other ACE-approved continuing education provider in your area, call ACE at (800) 825-3636 and ask for Professional Services, or visit our course locator at www.acefitness.org under "I'm Certified."

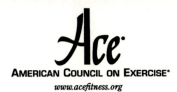

AMERICAN COUNCIL ON EXERCISE®
www.acefitness.org

YES, I would like to receive information on the following ACE certifications:
- ❏ Lifestyle & Weight Management Consultant
- ❏ Group Fitness Instructor
- ❏ Personal Trainer
- ❏ Clinical Exercise Specialist

Name _____
Address _____
City _____ State _____ ZIP _____
Home Phone (_____) _____
Work Phone (_____) _____
E-mail _____

Ace

AMERICAN COUNCIL ON EXERCISE®
www.acefitness.org

YES, I would like to receive information on the following ACE certifications:
- ❏ Lifestyle & Weight Management Consultant
- ❏ Group Fitness Instructor
- ❏ Personal Trainer
- ❏ Clinical Exercise Specialist

Name _____
Address _____
City _____ State _____ ZIP _____
Home Phone (_____) _____
Work Phone (_____) _____
E-mail _____

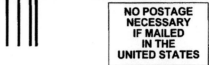

BUSINESS REPLY MAIL
FIRST-CLASS MAIL PERMIT NO. 22113 SAN DIEGO, CA

POSTAGE WILL BE PAID BY ADDRESSEE

AMERICAN COUNCIL ON EXERCISE
PO BOX 910449
SAN DIEGO CA 92191-9961

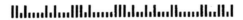

BUSINESS REPLY MAIL
FIRST-CLASS MAIL PERMIT NO. 22113 SAN DIEGO, CA

POSTAGE WILL BE PAID BY ADDRESSEE

AMERICAN COUNCIL ON EXERCISE
PO BOX 910449
SAN DIEGO CA 92191-9961

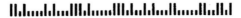